# THE FATTY LIVER CURE

## The Ultimate Principles to Reverse and Cure Fatty Liver

## &

## The Natural Liver Detox Cleanse

A Proven 7 Day Program To Cleanse Your Liver, Lose Weight And Reclaim Your Health

R. Huntington

© 2014 Copyright.
Text copyright reserved. R. Huntington

The contents of this book may not be reproduced, duplicated or transmitted without direct written permission from the author.

Disclaimer : all attempts have been made by the author to provide factual and accurate content. No responsibility will be taken by the author for any damages caused by misuse of the content described in this book. The content of this book has been derived from various sources. Please consult a licensed professional before attempting any techniques outlined in this book.

# Table of Contents

## Part 1 THE FATTY LIVER CURE   The Ultimate Principles to Reverse and Cure Fatty Liver ................. 1

Introduction ........................................................................... 2

Chapter 1: Fatty Liver and Its Causes ................................. 3

Chapter 2: Fatty Liver Symptoms and Signs ....................... 5

Chapter 3: Curing Fatty Liver Disease the Natural Way ....... 7

Chapter 4: Foods to Consume and Avoid with Fatty Liver .. 9

Chapter 5: Vitamins for Your Liver ................................... 11

Chapter 6: Avoiding Fatty Liver Disease with Exercise ...... 13

Chapter 7: Treating Fatty Liver with Herbs ........................ 15

Chapter 8: Why Liver Cleansing is Important .................... 16

Chapter 9: Cleansing Fatty Liver with Apple Cider Vinegar ............................................................................. 19

Chapter 10: The Liver Cleanse with grapefruit and olive oil ................................................................................... 22

Chapter 11: The Colon Cleanse ......................................... 25

Conclusion .......................................................................... 30

## Part 2 THE NATURAL LIVER DETOX CLEANSE   A Proven 7 Day Program To Cleanse Your Liver, Lose Weight and Reclaim Your ........................................ 31

Introduction ........................................................................ 32

Chapter 1 : The Liver Cleanse Explained .......................... 36

Chapter 2 : Your Shopping List For the Cleanse ................ 40

Chapter 3 : Preparing For the Cleanse ............................... 46

Chapter 4 : The Overnight Flush Step-by-Step .................. 50

Chapter 5 : The Results ............................................................ 55
Chapter 6 : After The Liver Cleanse ..................................... 58
Conclusion ................................................................................. 62
**Bonus ......................................................................... 63**

# Part 1
# THE FATTY LIVER CURE

## The Ultimate Principles to Reverse and Cure Fatty Liver

R. Huntington

# Introduction

I want to thank you and congratulate you for buying the book, *"The Natural Fatty Liver Cure: The Ultimate Principles to Reverse and Cure Fatty Liver."*

This book will teach you the different natural remedies to take away accumulated fat in your liver as well as remove harmful deposits in it such as gallbladder stones. It will also inform you the causes, symptoms and signs of fatty liver. These are information you should know of so that you would be able to determine if you are suffering from this condition. If you know what you are experiencing, you can prevent the disease from worsening and ultimately this book provides proven steps to cure fatty liver for life.

Thanks again for buying this book, I hope you enjoy it!

# Chapter 1:
# Fatty Liver and Its Causes

Fatty liver is a disease that happens when fat is accumulated in the cells of the liver organ.

This condition has two kinds and they are:

1. Alcoholic steatohepatitis

2. Nonalcoholic steatohepatitis or NASH.

Alcoholic steatohepatitis is the common of the two and this occurs when your liver is damaged due to excessive alcohol intake. NASH takes place when you are overweight or obese and you consume too much fatty and high-calorie food.

To diagnose if you have fatty liver disease, the doctor will ask you to undergo a blood test. The result shall be confirmed by either a CT scan or ultrasound. The blood test or even a routine exam will help inform your physician that you have an enlarged liver or an inflammation in your body. To remove other possible health problems, especially with your liver, your doctor may instruct you to go through more tests.

A fatty liver disease has two main causes and these are alcoholism and consumption of food that are fatty or high in calorie. People who are on a healthy diet rarely get this disease. Excessive calories can make fat build up in your liver and the latter will then have a hard time to perform its function which is to break fats down. Overconsumption of alcohol can also make fat accumulate in your liver. Genetics is also a possible cause.

There are times when malnourished people or those who quickly lose weight, especially after a weight-loss procedure, suffer from a fatty liver. Another theory by Ayurveda, iridology, Shiatsu and vibrational medicine practitioner Andreas Moritz is that a fatty liver can develop due to the formation of gallstones in the liver. It is falsely thought before that such stones only occur in the gallbladder but the truth is, most of them accumulate in the liver. When these stones are formed in the said organ, this can stop you from being healthy and energetic. Gallstones are actually a main reason why people become sick and do not recuperate easily and quickly from their sickness.

If you fail to treat liver diseases such as a fatty liver, this organ will become scarred and hardened and you will suffer from a serious condition called cirrhosis. Eventually, cirrhosis will result to liver failure. This condition has a few symptoms so you may not see signs of having it. If you are not aware about it, this can be very harmful and dangerous.

# Chapter 2:
# Fatty Liver Symptoms and Signs

Aside from the causes of a fatty liver mentioned in the last chapter which include alcoholism, an unhealthy diet, genetics, rapid weight loss and gallstones in the liver, it is vital to know what its symptoms and signs are so that you can find a treatment for it. Medical experts say a lot of sufferers experience only a few symptoms or signs, if none at all.

One of the symptoms of a fatty liver is a tummy pain which usually occurs above the abdomen at the right side of the area and under the rib cage. If the condition is not due to gas or gallstones, the pain will not be stabbing or sharp but rather, it is dull and has no obvious cause or pattern. This pain happens because the liver's surface stretches due to the fat cells building up. The inflammation and swelling in your liver will also cause pain.

Another sign of a fatty liver is skin pigmentation or darkening of the skin which is medically termed as acanthosis nigricans. The skin which is usually affected is the one surrounding the armpits and neck because these have a lot of sensitive glands. Acanthosis nigricans usually happens in children that have fatty liver not because of alcoholism. Their bodies try to combat fat accumulation frequently by creating more insulin from their armpit and neck glands.

The liver will at times change in shape and size because of the accumulation of fatty cells. Your physician can feel the liver when he presses some areas of the abdomen. Doctors usually do this in their routine checkups. When your liver has fatty tissue buildup, your doctor will feel it is bigger than normal. Aside from the size, your physician will also feel your liver's softened edge because of the cells having a lot of fat.

Another usual symptom of a fatty liver disease is constant exhaustion, according to medical experts. Usually, patients will not manifest this symptom till their liver is already noticeably enlarged. Malaise or weakness is also a symptom but this is frequently felt after getting a medical diagnosis.

A metabolic syndrome is linked with a fatty liver disease. This means if you have this liver disease, you may also suffer from metabolic syndrome.

If you are not aware you have the first symptoms of fatty liver and fat continues to build up in this organ, its tissues will become inflamed and scarred. This will make you incur more severe symptoms such as liver swelling, ascites or additional fluid in the middle of the abdominal tissues, menstrual problems if you are a female, swelling of breast tissues and inflated veins in your tummy or esophagus.

When fat accumulates in your liver, this is frequently associated or confused with other medical problems. Sufferers will experience diabetes, hypertension and obesity. If you are a fatty liver sufferer, you may also show signs and symptoms of diseases such as heart attack or failure, kidney failure or retinopathy which is the blood vessels in your eyes reacting abnormally.

Once you notice any of these symptoms in you, it is vital to see your doctor immediately.

# Chapter 3:
# Curing Fatty Liver Disease the Natural Way

When you are obese and are on a medically improper diet, this can cause a lot of health conditions like heart disease and hypertension. Aside from these, there is a great chance of acquiring a fatty liver which, if untreated, can permanently damage your liver. The good news is there are natural or home treatments which you can do so as to effectively overturn this disease. If you do not welcome prescription medications for fear of side effects, the natural way of curing fatty liver disease is ideal for you.

Obesity makes you prone to fatty liver so you need to decrease that risk by maintaining a good weight. Know your ideal weight from your doctor who will base it with your age, height and sex. Once you know what this is, try to achieve this weight and maintain it.

To lose weight, you have to change your eating patterns and lessen your consumption of sugars and foods that are high in fat and calories. Go for fruits and veggies because they will help decrease saturated fat in your meals and the accumulated fat in the liver. Also have more fish, nuts and whole grains in your diet and have snacks free of sugar such as yogurt.

Aside from a healthy diet, you should regularly work out so that your body fat is reduced and your blood triglycerides are lowered. When you are active, the fat buildup in your liver will be lessened and your fatty liver will be reversed. Try to exercise for half an hour to an hour thrice to five times per week.

Stay away from alcohol because excess intake will worsen fatty liver symptoms. Take healthy beverages instead such as fresh fruit and vegetable juices and green tea. Attempt to consume at least eight glasses of water every day so as to remove toxins from the organs of your body.

When you consume certain medications for a long time, this will damage your liver. If you already have fatty liver, such medications will slow down recovery and further destroy this organ. Always know the warnings on both prescription as well as non-prescription drugs and stay away from those which heighten the possibility of liver damage. You can speak to your physician about alternative medications for your health problems.

The following chapters will tell you of more natural remedies for a fatty liver disease.

# Chapter 4:
# Foods to Consume and Avoid with Fatty Liver

If you have fatty liver, you can avoid aggravating it by having dietary changes. Usually, a fatty liver disease is benign but if you ignore it and you do not take steps to prevent it, you may end up with cirrhosis and other diseases of the liver.

When on a diet to reverse fatty liver, you can consume plenty of organic vegetables as these have no fat and are enriched with vitamins. Always go for low or non-fat foods when treating this disease.

It is necessary to reduce the bad cholesterol or LDL in your blood as this in turn shall reduce the quantity of fat your liver absorbs. This shall then help decrease the liver's amount of work in removing such fats in your body. Consuming legumes and beans will help lower your LDL.

Taking fiber will also reduce LDL levels in your blood stream so take around 30 grams of it daily from fruits, veggies, supplements, flax seeds and whole grains. Whole grains are those that are not refined or processed so they do not have the identical amount of sugar found in processed cereals, white rice and white bread. Whole grains have natural nutrients like those found in whole wheat bread and brown rice so the body processes them slowly and discharges less fat via your blood stream.

To help in metabolizing fat, you can add choline, inositol and turmeric in your diet. You can also consume boldo tea as this toughens your gallbladder. Take dandelion and silymarin tea because they fortify the liver.

Aside from adding these specified foods in your diet, you also need to avoid certain foods so as to slow down the progress of your fatty liver disease or reverse it. Limit your consumption of refined carbohydrates taken from biscuits, breads, cakes, desserts, noodles, pasta, pastry and concentrated and processed sugar from candies, colas, sodas, ice cream, jellies, jams and powdered juice drinks. Concentrated sugar and refined carbohydrates inflame your body and disturb its blood sugar balance. Get rid of artificial sweeteners because they have additives and chemicals which compel your liver to function harder for digestion purposes.

Stay away from foods that are fatty and deep-fried like pork, red meat, butter, cheese, whole milk, coconut and palm oil, mayonnaise, pizza and French fries. Junk foods such as hamburgers, donuts and potato chips are strictly prohibited as they are made of partially hydrogenated or hydrogenated oils.

Stay away from turkey and chicken even if they are said to be healthy and enriched with lean protein because they do not emerge from sources that are organic. Non-organic poultry have additives like artificial grown hormones, antibiotics and steroids and the liver will have to function harder so as to digest them.

# Chapter 5:
# Vitamins for Your Liver

When you are suffering from liver diseases such as fatty liver, it is vital to take some vitamins to toughen up your liver.

One nutrient that strengthens the liver is the water-soluble Vitamin C as it enhances the function of this organ due to its regenerative qualities. You can get vitamin C from homemade lemon juice minus added sweeteners to help flush gallstones and toxins from both the gallbladder and liver. Aside from repairing damage done on the liver, this nutrient also fixes other tissues or organs inside the body. Eat citrus fruits and food containing Vitamin C like cabbage, spinach, broccoli, tomatoes, green peppers and strawberries. You can also take a supplement containing 500mg or more of this vitamin every day.

Another nutrient which can remove toxins from a slow liver is the beta carotene form of Vitamin A. This vitamin also enhances good skin as well as encourages healthy function of the organs. You should be careful in taking Vitamin A in the form of retinol because this is toxic to your liver when taken in big doses. Foods enriched with Vitamin A are apricots, beets, broccoli, carrots, fish, eggs, kale, peaches, squash and tomatoes.

You need to take Vitamin E as well because this protects Vitamin A and therefore helps enhance the function of the liver. If you combine these two together, you get a very powerful tonic which revitalizes and toughens your liver. You can get this nutrient from almonds, avocadoes, blueberries, cabbage, chard, collard, grains, spinach, sunflower seeds and walnuts.

To enhance liver decongestion, you will have to consume the B-vitamins like folic acid, B5, B6 and B12. The liver would easily perform its functions because these nutrients help it in breaking down the fats you consume. You need to consume a lot of B-vitamins foods or you can pop in a supplement containing of 50 grams or more of each of the B vitamins mentioned. Foods that have these nutrients are almonds, brewer's yeast, brown rice, pine nuts and sesame seeds.

Vitamin D is essential as well because it lowers body inflammations and therefore it helps maintain liver health. Your liver is so prone to inflammations by gallstones or other health problems. When you take this vitamin along with omega-3 fatty acids, this will heal your liver. You can find Vitamin D in bread, eggs, fish and milk, and omega-3 fatty acids from eggs, fish, fish oil and nuts. If your liver is healthy, it can, on its own, produce and use Vitamin D.

# Chapter 6:
# Avoiding Fatty Liver Disease with Exercise

According to a study made by a university in Missouri, you can actually avoid having fatty liver disease with exercise. This study showed that fatty liver disease and an inactive lifestyle are connected. It revealed that 100% of the rats that exercised everyday did not show signs or symptoms of this liver disease. Further, it revealed that in just a week of stopping daily physical activities, these rodents acquired fatty liver disease. The researchers then concluded that if you have enough quantity of exercise regularly, you can avoid this harmful disease which does not usually produce visible symptoms.

You do not have to pay a membership free in a gym to get daily exercise. You can work out for half an hour by walking or jogging around the neighborhood. You can also do aerobics at home in front of a DVD showing different aerobic workouts. Take a dip in the community swimming pool and swim around for an hour. You can also dance to your favorite tune in the comfort of your own room or lift those weights in your home gym. You can also wash your care as this can burn down calories.

If bad weather stops you from getting regular workouts, you can exercise at home by jumping rope, doing yoga, lifting heavy books, running up and down the stairs or dancing with your family. If you have the money, enroll in a gym or you can purchase weights, an elliptical trainer or a treadmill you can use during a gloomy weather.

If you have a BMI or body mass index more than 25, you will need a tougher exercise and diet plan so as to get rid of your excess weight. Try to burn off a couple of pounds week with healthy eating and regular physical activities.

Be consistent in working out. In the study mentioned, the rats stopped being physically active for a week and they immediately got fatty liver disease. Most of the time, people exercise in the first month but afterwards, they gradually stop working out. To be inspired to exercise regularly, you can work out with a friend or have a personal trainer who shall monitor your progress and keep you right on track.

Another way to motivate you in exercising regularly is to perform activities you enjoy doing and add variety to them. If you like what you are doing, it would be a lot easier for you to be consistent. You can join a running group or any sports team for that matter. You not only exercise but you also have an active social life as well.

# Chapter 7:
# Treating Fatty Liver with Herbs

The initial stage of liver damage is a fatty liver disease and this may be followed by cirrhosis or liver fibrosis. Natural remedies for this disease include the use of certain herbs which help reverse damage done on the liver.

One of the herbs that help nourish the liver and make it work properly is barberry. You can take 400mg of barberry supplement every day. Be careful though because taking too much of it promotes toxicity. Pregnant women are advised against taking this herb because it can lead to a miscarriage.

Another herb that helps digest food and enhance the liver is Cascara Sagrada. You can take 1ml of this herb daily in tincture form. Pregnant women should not take this herb. When you frequently take it though, it can make you suffer from diarrhea. Ask your doctor the time frame of taking this herb.

A very potent cleanser for the liver is dandelion. You can take this raw or in supplement or tincture form. If you take it in tincture form, consume 5 ml to 10 ml of it daily. The side effects of this herb though are dermatitis and digestive problems.

For your liver to properly function and digest food, you should take gentian root. You can take this as a supplement at 3 grams to 6 grams a day. It has side effects which include mild headaches.

You can also take golden seal which cleanses and purifies your liver. Consume 4 grams to 6 grams of the supplement form. Pregnant women should not consume this because it can cause nervousness and digestive problems.

# Chapter 8:
# Why Liver Cleansing is Important

Of all the organs, it is the liver which directly controls the development and performance of all the body cells. When the cells grow abnormally, malfunction or become deficient, this is because of the poor performance of the liver. Due to its unique design, your liver may look as if it works normally through blood values that are balanced even if it has lost 60% of its initial effectiveness. This can deceive you and your doctor. Most of the health diseases originate from the liver. To help prevent this, liver cleansing is needed.

When you liver cleanse, this means you decongest your gallbladder and liver bile ducts so that all your body cells will receive more oxygen and nutrients, get rid of metabolic waste products as well as sustain good communication links among your body parts, endocrine system and nervous system.

Liver cleansing will help remove gallstones in your liver. It is necessary to take away these stones because they contribute to almost any kind of disease. When you take away these stones via liver cleansing, you will permanently have vital health.

Many neuropathic physicians suggest that prior to doing a liver cleansing program, preparatory work has to be done initially so that the process will be more effective. You have to undergo a parasite or colon cleanse one to three months so that excess waste stuck on your colon walls will be removed from your body. To do a colon cleanse, you should have a diet with just raw fruits and veggies. Processed foods must be avoided. You can also find effective colon cleansing programs online or at health food shops in your locality. Once you have a clean colon, your liver will be able to respond effectively with a cleansed intestinal system. After establishing three bowel movements per day, you can now start liver cleansing.

You need to stop consuming alcohol once you have cleansed your colon. You should also eat foods which help in liver cleansing such as oats, garlic, onions, cinnamon, beans, dark green leafy greens, flaxseed and turmeric. Stay away from foods that are processed or not grown organically. You should have more citrus fruits in your diet like papayas and oranges as they help maintain a good liver.

If you are pregnant, never undergo a liver cleansing. Do not do this program if you are very sick or if you suffer from constipation. Young children should never do a liver cleanse.

Perform a liver cleanse on a weekend because you are not aware of your body's reaction the first time you do this. You may have to urinate or defecate frequently in a day so you need to say at home for this. Your body will eliminate toxins and gallstones via your bowels. There are those who feel exhausted or sick during their initial cleansing program because they are removing toxins from their body very rapidly. The toxins make you feel light-headed, weak or tired while they go out of the body.

When liver cleansing, there are some things you need and these include certain herbs, Epsom salts, lemons and an effective juicer. The herbs you may need are milk thistle and black walnut hull in tincture forms. If you do not want to make your own tonic, visit a health food shop and ask if they have liver cleansing products.

If you suffer from grave digestive health issues, a naturopathic doctor will have to monitor you while you are on a liver cleanse. You will see gallstones coming out of your body as you do this program. These are just small stones but there are times that they can be quite big and may irritate your other organs and result to an obstruction. Make sure to closely monitor yourself when you are cleansing and should you suffer severe pain, you have to go to your doctor immediately.

Once you have properly cleansed your colon and your liver, you will be more energetic and your extra weight will be shed off. Additionally, your gall stones will also be eliminated. Your body will be able to function well as one harmonious unit and you will have a healthier life.

# Chapter 9:
# Cleansing Fatty Liver with Apple Cider Vinegar

One of the popular natural detoxifiers of the body is vinegar and of all its types, it is apple cider vinegar considered the most potent and effective to eliminate fat surrounding and inside your liver. This is because this vinegar is said to be the least acidic of them all and is gentle on your digestive tract once it goes inside the body. Over time, it also breaks down all the fatty deposits and promotes a healthy bladder, kidney and liver. If you are suffering from hypertension, this vinegar can also serve as a blood thinner. Because it is acidic, it kills bacteria and lessens liver inflammation and irritation. Prior to using this kitchen product for the removal of fatty deposits in your liver, consult your doctor first.

Raw and unfiltered apple cider vinegar can be consumed in different ways to eliminate fatty deposits in your liver. After a month of using this product, you should go to your doctor again and check your liver condition to check if it is still enlarged and inflamed. If this is the case, you will need to cleanse again for another month. Always brush your teeth or utilize an oral mouthwash so that your tooth enamel will be safeguarded from erosion from the vinegar.

The first method of using apple cider vinegar involves shaking the bottle so that all its contents will be equally distributed inside and that no sedimentation is left at the bottom. Get eight ounces of water and mix in one tablespoon of this vinegar. Drink this tonic thrice to six times every day prior to taking your meals so as to break down fats you consumed and enhance digestive processes.

The second method is not as acidic as the first method because you have less vinegar to consume. It is also sweeter. First shake the bottle containing your vinegar for equal dispersion of the contents inside and no sedimentation will lie at the bottom. Get one glass of water and mix one tablespoon each of apple cider vinegar and honey. This shall sweeten your tonic. Drink this tonic twice per day by drinking half of it in the morning while the other half must be consumed in the evening.

Have a liver detoxification cleanse twice a year. You can do one in autumn and the other one during spring. Eat a light meal with foods that are easy to digest on the night prior to your detox. You can have fish and steamed veggies. On the day you will detox, have a liquid fast wherein you will only consume broths, green tea, veggie juices, apple juice and other healthy liquids. When you wake up, take your apple cider tonic as prescribed in the first method. Increase the strength of this tonic by adding a tablespoon of the vinegar.

Seven days after your detox, consume 100% fresh fluids such as fruits, veggies, legumes, lean meats, non-fat dairy products and whole grains. You may experience lightheadedness, nausea and headaches as you fast because the toxins are already being eliminated from the body. While you are liver cleansing, you should also do some light activities, such as stretching and walking, and get some air and sunshine.

Aside from the two methods mentioned earlier, you can also have a liver cleansing tea from apple cider vinegar. Just mix a couple of tablespoons of this vinegar in a cup of boiling or hot water and then sweeten this with maple syrup or honey. Every day, drink a cup of this tea.

Apple cider vinegar and honey tonics can also aid in weight loss when you take them half an hour before your meals. You will feel full with this tonic and your appetite will be controlled. In addition, this tonic will help burn fat because apple cider vinegar and honey have fat-burning properties.

After you have taken apple cider vinegar, make sure you eat something immediately as there are individuals who suffer mild nausea when they take this alone. Never take undiluted apple cider vinegar as this can destroy your esophagus, tooth enamel and other parts of the digestive tract. If you suffer from osteoporosis or low levels of blood potassium, do not take this vinegar. If you are suffering from diabetes, you should ask your doctor first before using this product because this may affect your insulin levels.

## Chapter 10:
## The Liver Cleanse with grapefruit and olive oil

There is one liver cleanse system which theorizes that your body becomes more energized if your liver is healthy and is in optimal condition. Based on proven steps this week-long super-cleanse eliminates hundreds of tiny gallstones which have built up in his liver over the years.

If you have stones in your gallbladder and liver, you may experience the following symptoms:

- Alzheimer's disease
- Asthma
- Brain disorders
- Cancer
- Chronic fatigue
- Constipation
- Depression
- Difficulty in breathing
- Digestive disorders
- Food cravings
- Gout
- Hemorrhoids
- Insomnia

- Nightmares
- Obesity
- Puffy eyes or skin
- PMS
- Sciatica
- Scoliosis

In this chapter, you will find a seven-day liver cleanse plan. Make sure you have one and a half gallons of apple juice water, four tablespoons of Epsom salt, half a cup of cold-pressed extra virgin olive oil and two-thirds glass freshly-squeezed lemon or grapefruit juice mixed with orange juice.

For the first six days of your liver cleanse, you need to consume 32 ounces of apple juice daily. It has malic acid which softens the gallstones so that they can easily pas while doing this six-day juice cleansing, you shouldn't eat protein rich food Do not take any medication, supplements or vitamins if possible. This cleanse must be done on weekends or at a time when you will just be staying at home for the whole day because you will experience some discomfort.

Upon the sixth day of consuming apple juice, drink it in the morning and eat a light meal ( rice with carrots) about 1:00P.M.. It is after 1:30 P.M. when you can only drink water.

Mix four tablespoons of Epsom salt and 32 ounces of water and pour this mixture in a clean jar. Drink eight ounces of this mixture at 6:00 P.M.. This can have a nasty taste so you can try pinching your nose when consuming it. Make sure you stay close to a toilet.

At around 8:00 P.M., you need to drink eight more ounces of the mixture.

At 9:45 P.M you have to squeeze and mix together your citrus fruits and half a cup of your extra virgin olive oil. After another 15 minutes, you have to quickly drink this mixture and then lie down on your back. Make sure your head is propped over the abdomen. You can also lie down on the right side with the knees pulled to the head. For not less than 20 minutes, lie down perfectly still.

The following morning at around 6:00 AM, you should consume eight ounces of your salt water mixture. After two hours, at 8:00 AM consume the remaining eight ounces of salt water.

Rest throughout the day but always maintain an erect position because this will make the gallbladder stones pass smoothly.
At around 10:30 A.M., you can begin eating after initially drinking fruit juice. You can eat fruit and then eventually add heavier foods all through the day. Make sure though to keep it light.

It is recommended to perform an enema or a colon cleanse a few days following your liver cleanse so that all the stones come out and will not rot in your colon. In addition, it is recommended to do a kidney cleanse prior to or following four to five cleanses because the kidney may be filled up with toxins. One way of kidney cleansing is taking water every morning that has one teaspoon of dissolved Epsom salt in it for a period of two weeks.

# Chapter 11:
# The Colon Cleanse

Prior to and after performing liver cleansing, you also need to cleanse your colon. People today consume so much processed foods that are deprived of most of their natural form, fiber and nutrients. Because of this, the muscles surrounding your colon find it difficult to transport the food mass that are partially digested. These substances may stay in your colon for a long time and will soon become drier and harder. If you have waste such as bacteria, dead cellular tissue, hardened mucus, impacted feces, and other toxic substances built up and trapped in your colon, they may go inside your blood and lymph streams. You will then feel ill, sluggish, or tired. You may suffer from colon-related diseases such as backaches, bloating, bad breath, constipation, body odor, diarrhea, nausea, headaches, sinusitis, dizziness, ear and eye problems, and other nervous system disorders. Eventually, you may suffer from colon cancer.

Ideally, a colon cleanse must be done on the 6th day of the liver cleanse and within three days after every liver cleanse. If you do not clean out your colon, you may have toxemia and plenty of other adverse effects which can offset the benefits of liver cleaning. Do not perform a liver cleanse if you will not clean your colon.

If there is something in your colon which constricts or congests, your gallbladder will not readily open when you are liver cleansing. Even your liver's bile ducts may not open or relax easily because of congestion, blockage or sticky stool in your colon or because of constipation. On the colon walls are reflex points linked to your gallbladder and liver and they are the ones that send signals to these organs not to secrete bile as they are not prepared to welcome new food. These reflex points urge the body not to eat or to stimulate your appetite. Once the bile is absent, your appetite is suppressed. The body then signals the brain and your senses not to eat and therefore, not to cleanse. If you do a liver cleanse, it will not be successful if the colon is not itself cleansed.

However, if you do not colon cleanse yet you do a liver cleanse and gallbladder stones are passed, there is a possibility that these stones might get caught somewhere in your large intestine. If you do not perform a colon cleanse after the liver cleanse, these stones have a great chance of getting caught in your colon and will eventually disintegrate.

The stones that usually come out of your gallbladder and liver are not calcium stones. Instead, they are soft, fatty, oily, waxy and putty-like because they are composed of fats clogged up in your liver's bile ducts. The moment they come out, a huge amount of toxins is released in your colon. Bacteria inside the colon decompose these toxins and these cannot be discarded via enemas, colema or colonics.

The toxins released in your colon will go into your blood stream and produce toxic effects. Your blood then goes back into your liver and the possibility of producing new stones is high because these toxins go into your large intestines.

If there are only a few stones left in your colon after liver cleansing, you need to undergo a colon cleanse in two or three days time. The kind of colon cleanse you need to perform should not be the oral form because magnesium oxide or Epsom salts are not enough. You will need to undergo an enema or a colema which is a water-based flushing procedure.

If you will do an enema, the water you use must go way up the opposite side and into your ascending colon. A single enema is insufficient because you need to do three consecutive enemas.

You need to release everything inside till nothing comes out anymore and until the water reaches the starting part of your colon in the part that ascends. Such a process will ensure that your liver cleanse is safe, you will have a balanced system and you will not be contaminated by the toxins of the trapped gallbladder stones in your colon.

Another type of colon cleansing is colon hydrotherapy which is also known as colonic or colonic irrigation. It is a very effective way of cleansing your colon and in just a brief period, trapped waste in whatever amount that has accumulated for years will be eliminated. This process takes 40 to 50 minutes and around two to six liters of clean, boiled water will be used to softly flush your colon. During the colonic, a gentle abdominal massage is done so as to loosen old deposits of fecal matter and mucus that have hardened. Once they are loosened, water will flush them out.

Aside from removing damaging toxic wastes, a colonic hydrates and revitalizes the muscles of your colon. The continuous passage and discharge of water enhances the peristaltic action of the colon and minimizes the travel time of toxic matter. A colonic also restores the natural shape of your colon and rouses the reflex points connecting your colon to all your body parts. It can separate waste and its old crusted layers from the walls of your colon. It therefore allows better hydration of your colon and enhanced water absorption. For these benefits to happen, you need to do not less than two or three colonic sessions.

When you are undergoing a colonic, you might feel slightly uncomfortable, especially when there are huge amounts of toxic waste that come off your intestinal walls and go to your rectum. Afterwards, though, you will feel light and clean and your mind will be clearer. Whatever discomfort you will feel will be offset by these benefits you will have later on.

A colonic can help fight your emotional problems. Your transverse colon goes through your solar plexus, the emotional center of your body. Almost all of a person's undigested or unresolved emotional problems are in your solar plexus and they cause the muscles of the colon to tighten. Because of this, you will suffer from constipation and a slow bowel movement. When you undergo a colonic irrigation, the physical obstruction in your colon will be cleared and the tension which causes your emotional distress will be released.

When your stomach is empty for two to three hours after you have eaten, perform a colonic cleanse. Afterwards, you should consume one to two glasses of water and then after thirty minutes, consume one fruit or a glass of fresh fruit juice. Your first couple of meals must be light after the cleanse. You will see that your bowel movement will be naturally restored in a couple of days. Should restoration of bowel movement take longer than that, it means your colon has so much waste that has accumulated for many years. You will then have to undergo more colonics until everything has been removed.

There are many kinds of colony hydrotherapy systems that are now being used. Professional colonic therapists get their training from different sources. You may have to prepare some amount for this because a one-hour session usually costs $50-$75.

To do a colon cleanse, you should have a diet with just raw fruits and vegetables. Processed foods must be avoided. You can also find effective colon cleansing programs online or at health food shops in your community. Once you have a clean colon, your liver will be able to respond effectively with a cleansed intestinal system. After establishing three bowel movements per day, you can now start liver cleansing.

You need to stop consuming alcohol once you have cleansed your colon. You should also eat foods which help in liver cleansing such as oats, garlic, onions, cinnamon, beans, dark green leafy vegetables, flaxseed, and turmeric. Stay away from foods that are processed or not grown organically. You should have more citrus fruits in your diet like papayas and oranges as they help maintain a good liver.

# Conclusion

Thank you again for buying this book!

I hope this book was able to help you to learn more about curing fatty liver and the wonders of alternative treatments.

At the same time I hope that this book was able to help you better understand your role in curing your own fatty liver, and that having a healthy lifestyle that includes the right diet and ample amount of exercise are very important to cure and prevent fatty liver.

I hope this book served as a guide for healthier living.


Thank you and good luck!

# Part 2
# THE NATURAL LIVER DETOX CLEANSE

## A Proven 7 Day Program To Cleanse Your Liver, Lose Weight and Reclaim Your

R. Huntington

# Introduction

How many times have you woken up not feeling quite as well as you'd like but not quite ill enough to go to the doctor? How many times have you suddenly felt unexplained headaches, abdominal or back aches whose symptoms develop almost as fast as they disappeared? Do you have food allergies that you've just recently developed? Have you tried to lose weight yet the pounds don't seem to drop off despite the fact that you're doing everything right? Do you feel unexplainably tired, bloated or depressed?

Maybe that's your liver's way of telling you that it needs to be cleansed.

The liver is the largest organ in the body and one of the most important. It purifies the blood. It produces hormones necessary for reproductive health. It produces bile necessary for digestion. It controls the growth and function of each cell in the body. Any food, beverage or toxins that enter your body whether through eating, inhalation or via your skin MUST pass through the liver where they are either converted into enzymes and nutrients the body needs to properly function or eliminated.

Because it comes into contact with literally everything that passes through the body, it is no wonder that the liver is also one of the most susceptible organs to damage. Nature was kind enough to make the liver one of the few organs of the body capable of regenerating themselves. However it is not indestructible! When there are too many 'bad' substances coming in, the liver becomes overwhelmed leading to slowdown, scarring and reduction in its ability to perform its functions.

What exactly are these 'bad' substances?

Let's take an example of the food we eat. Our forefathers were masters of health. Food was only eaten when it was needed and even then eaten in its purest form – from the earth to the stomach. However these days the methods of processing food for human consumption have been over-complicated in an effort to make food more 'flavorful'. There is no generation that has eaten as much fatty food, spiced food or genetically modified food as ours. It is no wonder that we are constantly trying to deal with the plagues of obesity, cancers and other complications that can be directly linked to our compromised diets.

The problem with all this fat and flavor is that the liver is now being forced to process toxins it was not originally programmed to deal with. Because it cannot process them out of the system fast enough, these toxins accumulate and lead to the formation of gallstones (chunks of hardened bile and other trapped organic and inorganic substances) which then clog the liver and interfere with the filtering process.

Once your liver is obstructed like this, it hard for the whole body to function well. Your digestive system is affected and it is now much harder for the right nutrients to be processed and the harmful ones to be eliminated. Your respiratory system is affected because the blood purification has been compromised which means red blood cells have a harder time carrying oxygen and carbon-dioxide isn't being eliminated from the system effectively enough. Your reproductive system is distressed because the hormones it needs to function are over-produced. You age faster because your cells aren't regenerating as fast as they should. Basically, your whole body begins to fall apart.

It is heartening to see the recent worldwide interest in better health and the recent movements to bring back healthy foods to our tables. It means that our livers will have less toxicity to deal with. However, we still have one problem. A healthy lifestyle will only prevent the formation of more gallstones. What about the ones that have already been formed?

Once gallstones have been formed, they aren't just going to disappear because you've suddenly decided to become healthy. And while they are there they aren't just going to be silent investors in your body. They will continue to clog the system and release toxins that compromise the liver's functions. Sure with a better diet they may eventually start to breakdown, but the process may not be fast enough for you to experience the benefits of your new healthy choices.

Hence the Natural Liver Detox Cleanse!

The Liver Cleanse is a way of decongesting your liver, the bile ducts that are critical to its functions and your colon immediately. With a process that only lasts from the evening of one day to the morning of the next, you can get rid of the gallstones obstructing your system. And yes, you still get your regular eight hour sleep.

Ingredients introduced to the system during the flush will soften and breakdown the gallstones. They'll dilate and oil the bile ducts to ensure the now softened gallstones travel through the body with as little drama as possible. It is an easy, pain-free and safe process that will leave you feeling like a new person.

The effects of the Liver Cleanse are almost immediate. You will feel the immediate rejuvenation of your system. Your digestive system will be cleaned out. Your blood will be purified. The hormones in your body will be balanced better and your cells will be able to regenerate faster. You will look, feel and be better!

If that isn't an excellent reason to try out the Liver Cleanse, I don't know what is.

In this book you will learn;

- How and why the Liver Cleanse works
- What ingredients you need for to successfully cleanse your liver
- How to prepare for the Liver Cleanse
- How to do the overnight Liver Cleanse on your own in the comfort of your own house
- The results to expect
- The long-term lifestyle changes you can make that will prevent the formation of future obstructions to your body.

My hope is that by the end of this book you will be just as healthy as many people who have already gone through this Natural Liver Detox Cleanse and improved their health through it.

Good luck!

# Chapter 1 :
# The Liver Cleanse Explained

The mechanics of the Liver Cleanse are not complicated. The process is designed to flush out gallstones and any other accumulated organic and inorganic substances from the liver and the colon. Once these toxicities are removed from the system, the liver will be able to function better and thus influence the better functioning of all other systems within your body.

There are four main elements critical to the success of the Liver Flush, namely;

- Malic Acid

- A clean diet pre-cleanse

- Epsom Salt

- Oil

- Citrus

The Malic Acid acts on the mainly alkali based gallstones, softening them and even breaking some of them down for ease of passage down the colon. Because it is not an instant process, juices containing Malic acid are introduced into the system in small portions starting from six days before the actual overnight flush to commence the softening. While the Malic Acid is acting on gallstones, you need to minimize the formation of new ones and this can only be done by maintaining a clean diet the six days prior to the actual overnight cleanse.

On the evening of the actual cleanse, Epsom salt will be introduced into the system. Unlike other salts, Epsom is magnesium based rather than sodium based increasing its capability to dilate the bile ducts and sphincter muscles. This makes the passage of the gallstones much easier. It also encourages bowel movement pre-cleanse to eliminate any other obstructions that are not gallstones.

For the actual cleanse, a blend of Extra Virgin Oil and citrus fruit juice is taken in. The Epsom salt has already cleared the pathway but the oil is necessary to trigger bile release essential to forcing the stones to begin their movement through the bile ducts to the colon. That last shot of malic acid courtesy of the citrus fruit blended with the oil will soften any stones that still need coercing. The oil coating the marble like substances will make the process smooth and prevent any damage of the ducts because of scrapping.

Once the gallstones are out, you're home free and should begin to feel the benefits of a cleaner system.

**WHEN SHOULD YOU DO IT**

The overnight flush is best done over the weekend. Over the weekend you are under less pressure from the daily chores of life and can concentrate on your health. Because the overnight flush requires six days of preparation for the over haul by introducing Malic acid to your system and keeping your diet clean, it is best to reserve a week when you will be sure there will be no temptation to eat unhealthy foods. Avoid weeks that have holidays, family gatherings, office parties or any other events requiring interaction with fatty or over-processed food.

Children as young as nine years-old and adults as old as ninety years-old have successfully undergone the liver flush, so if you're between these ages and relatively healthy, it is okay to do the Liver Cleanse. If you're taking any food supplements that are not critical to your health, plan to discontinue them during the week preceding the overnight flush. Your system needs to be in as natural a state as possible.

Get yourself weighed and your BMI measured by a certified medical practitioner before you make the decision to do a Liver Cleanse. You need to be as healthy as possible for this process. If you're overweight it's okay to do the flush but if you are underweight, your first priority should be to get to a healthy weight first.

For women, the overnight flush is best done after or before your menstrual cycle – not during. Your cycle is already a cleansing process and having two going on at the same time will stress your system unnecessarily. Besides that the Liver Cleanse is a much more comfortable process when done on its own.

If you're just coming out of chemotherapy or any other kind of cancer treatment you need to wait for eight or ten months to elapse after your treatment to try the Liver Cleanse. The reason for this is because your bile ducts are already weakened due to the heavy toxins introduced during chemo. The vigorous nature of the Liver Cleanse may only worsen this condition so you need to wait till your body can handle the cleanse before you attempt it.

**WHO SHOULD NOT DO IT**

If you're taking any drugs – prescription or nonprescription – do not attempt the Liver Cleanse. There has been no real test to determine what reaction the ingredients in the cleansing blends would have when mixed with other drugs and the subsequent side-effects. It is best not to do the Liver Cleanse at all and be safe. There are long-term ways to cleanse your liver including introducing a morning glass of juiced lemon into your diet that are moderate and will not stress your system.

If you feel the Liver Cleanse is something you really need to clean your system, then you need to talk to your doctor who will then determine if it is safe for you to attempt it. Even then, people with any kind of bowel disorder e.g. Crohn's Disease and Hernia should not attempt the cleanse at all.

Pregnant, Planning-to-be-Pregnant and Nursing women shouldn't attempt the Liver Cleanse. Your body needs to conserve all its energy for the reproduction system. Diverting it to the digestive system will only stress you. Furthermore, there is no way to know what effect the ingredients may have on your hormones. Instead concentrate on maintaining a healthy lifestyle during this period in your life. The Liver Cleanse isn't going anywhere.

# Chapter 2 :
# Your Shopping List For the Cleanse

For a successful Liver Cleanse, you're going to need to have a few things on the ready. Below is a handy list of everything you'll need and in what measures.

**THE JUICE**

Before the gallstones (along with other toxins) can be flushed out of the system, they need to be broken down into smaller pieces that will travel easier down the colon. Malic acid has been shown to be extremely effective in doing this. When taken over a period of time, it reacts with the alkali in the gallstones thus softening and/or breaking them down.

You have several options; the first of which is apple juice. You're going to need to drink 32oz (1 liter) each day, for at least six days so make sure to get enough (about 6 liters). The best option for you is to just buy the apples and then juice them at home yourself each day. However, commercial apple juice will work just as well. You just need to check the labels to make sure that you are getting 100% apple juice.

You may also choose to use sour/tart cherry juice. It is a less sugary option that diabetics and hypoglycemics will appreciate. Apart from aiding in the liver cleanse, it also comes with added benefits. If you've got joint inflammations, cherry juice has been shown to alleviate the inflammations. It is also known to lower the blood pressure, improve blood circulation within the body and prevent tumor growths. Sour/tart cherry juice contains four times as much malic acid as what is found in apple juice. Therefore just get a quarter as much (8oz/240ml for each day).

If neither apple juice nor sour/tart cherry juice is available to you, try unsweetened cranberry juice. Because it is unsweetened, you only need half as much cherry juice as apple juice. Get 16oz (500ml) of cherry juice for each day. You'll need to mix it with some water (8-16oz) to dilute the tartness.

## THE SALT

To help with the cleansing of the colon, you're going to need a lot of Magnesium Sulphate also known as Epsom salt. Epsom salt is critical for three main functions – to contract the gallbladder and thus force out gallstones, to widen the bile ducts and prompt release of more bile and to relax the sphincter for a more comfortable passing of the gallstones.

There has been a lot of hullabaloo about Epsom salt with people spreading a lot of myths about its dangers. Generally Epsom salt has no side-effects on healthy people. The only circumstances when you need to avoid it is when you're breast feeding or pregnant or you're taking prescription or non-prescription drugs - all conditions that bar you from doing the liver cleanse anyway.

You need at least 4 tablespoons of Epsom salt that you can find in any drug store or your local natural foods' store. It is extremely rare for someone to be allergic to magnesium or sulphate, however if you are consider using Magnesium Citrate instead in the exact same quantity.

## THE OIL

You're going to need 4oz (120ml) of Extra Virgin Oil. Oil is a critical component of the overnight of the cleanse. Without it, the process may cause spasms of pain because the bile ducts aren't well lubricated. With it, the process is much smoother and your sleep will not be disrupted by the cleanse.

The problem with olive oil is that there are so many brands out there with misleading labels. Many say they are 100% Extra virgin oil when they've been blended with other oils like soy or canola oil which will compromise the Liver Cleanse. You need real 100% Extra Virgin Oil. The way to know that you have the genuine thing is to first concentrate your spending on brands imported from Italy, Greece or Spain. They are relatively expensive than normal brands but this is because they are often the real virgin oil. Even for these brands check the color of the oil in the bottle. It should be greenish in color.

There are some people who cannot tolerate Extra Virgin Oil. If you have problems with it consider replacing it with Macadamia oil, cold-pressed grape seed-oil or sun-flower oil. However please note that Extra Virgin oil is really your best option if you want this process to be successful. By all means avoid processed oils like soy, canola or corn oil.

**CITRUS**

During the overnight cleanse, the oil will be mixed with citrus that will provide the malic acid needed to soften the gallstones as they begin to move through the bile ducts. Any citrus fruit will do. You can choose to use fresh grapefruit or you can use a combination of orange and lemon juice. You need enough citrus to squeeze out at least 6oz (180ml) of juice.

If you can't tolerate the grapefruit juice or the orange and lemon blend, then you can just use apple juice or tart cherry juice. However they are not ideal options since they do not act as fast as citrus does within the time needed for it to start acting on the gallstones.

## WHOLE GRAINS, FRUITS & VEGETABLES

For at least a week before the overnight liver cleanse, you need to keep your diet as healthy as possible. The best way to do this is to incorporate into your diet a lot of whole grains, fresh fruits, vegetables and 'good' fats while eliminating 'bad' fats found mainly in meat and dairy products.

There are countless fruits and vegetables available out there depending on what season you are in but do remember to add to your shopping list fruits like apples, bananas and avocados that keep you satisfied for longer. Green vegetables like kales and spinach are an absolute must as they contain nutrients that aid the digestive system in its functions.

Replace your regular coffee with a ginger-lemon-warm water blend. Ginger will activate your metabolism, lemon will stimulate bowel movement and the warm water will hydrate your body. Just half a lemon squeezed into a warm glass of water and a half inch knob of ginger root grated into the blend should be enough to help you get even more health benefits than your usual coffee. If you must sweeten the blend then use honey instead of processed sugar. While honey contains just as many calories as processed sugar, it is kinder to the system in terms of the nutrients it adds to your body and it is also natural

Replace white grains (e.g. white rice, white bread) with whole grains (e.g. oats, brown rice, whole wheat) as they will keep you fuller for longer and are also easier on your digestive system. During this time, you need to eliminate animal products including meat, fish, poultry, eggs and dairy products from your diet as well as fried foods. Even just changing the kind of oil you go with from regular oil to Extra virgin olive oil will help your system prepare itself for restoration. It is also good practice for the lifestyle changes you will need to make after the cleanse.

Stock your pantry with enough of these healthy foods to last at least nine days (six days before the overnight cleanse and three days after the cleanse).

## OPTIONAL INGREDIENTS

### Aloe Vera Juice.

A few people who underwent the cleanse reported nausea the morning after the overnight cleanse. Just in case you experience it, it's handy to have some aloe vera juice on hand. It will ease the nausea and settle your stomach.

### Lemons.

Even if you chose to use grapefruit for your overnight cleanse, you still should have some lemons on hand. Some people have a hard time drinking the Espom salt and water mixture. For these people adding some lemon to a bit of water and sipping it between drinking the Epsom salt and water mixture helped make the process much smoother.

### Honey.

During the actual overnight cleanse, you will be required to drink a blend of Extra Virgin oil and citrus. Most people will not have a hard time taking in the blend. However for those who do, taking a bit of honey in between the gulps will help ease the process.

# EQUIPMENT

## Measuring Jar.

A lot of the Ingredients needed during the cleanse require measuring to exact proportions. Having a measuring jar on hand will make it that much easier to be accurate with your quantities and thus ensure the success of the process.

## Sealed Containers/Bottles.

Blends like the Epsom salt and water mixture will require storing overnight. Storing them out in the open may lead to contamination and compromise your liver cleans process. Using sealed bottles or containers will help prevent this from happening.

## Glass Jar with Lid.

The oil and citrus blend will need to be shaken so that it mixes well. Oil tends to cling to plastic so it wouldn't make a good container for the mixture. The lid is to prevent it from spilling.

## Water Enema.

It is recommended that you do a colon cleanse two to three days before and after the Liver Cleanse. However if you choose not to do it, keep a water enema on hand just in case, you have a problem releasing the gallstones.

# Chapter 3 :
# Preparing For the Cleanse

Before you can do the overnight liver cleanse, you need at least six days of preparation. These six days are critical for the break down and dissolving of the gallstones into smaller pieces that can pass through the bile ducts easily. Already we've said the overnight flush is best done over the weekend. Therefore your Day One should either be on a Sunday or a Monday. This way your overnight flush will fall smack on the weekend (Friday or Saturday night)!

**DAY 0**

This is the day you're basically preparing for the whole process that will lead to the overnight flush. Your first task is to read through this whole guide and make sure that you understand what the liver cleanse is all about as well as the schedule you'll be required to keep to ensure that your cleanse is successful.

You also need to collect all the ingredients necessary for the Liver Cleanse. Make sure you have your juice with malic acid, Epsom salt, Extra Virgin oil and citrus as well as the optional ingredients that will help you out in case you have difficulty drinking the blends. Remember to stock your pantry with enough healthy foods (whole grains, fruits and vegetables) to last you at least the next ten days.

This is also your chance to prepare yourself mentally, not just for the overnight cleanse but for the six days before then. For some people, healthy eating may not have been a priority before the flush. However for the flush to be effective, you'll need to maintain a healthy diet for at least six days before the flush. This will require some self-control on your part that can only be brought about by real commitment to the process.

Visualize all the benefits you're going to get from your liver being clean. Your digestive system will be more revitalized which means those pesky abdominal pains will be no more. Without gallstones, it will be much easier for you to maintain your weight. Your skin will be clearer and your thinking will be clearer. Just thinking of the immense benefits of a flushed liver should be enough to help you commit. Plan to reward yourself as soon as you successfully finish the flush. It can be a book, a trip to the newest movie or a vacation, just to congratulate yourself on sticking to the process and following it step-by-step.

You also need to get support from the people living with you. The people who are closest to you should know that you will be undergoing a health process in the course of the week. Maybe you can even convince them to go through the Liver Cleanse with you. This way it won't just be you who's healthy – but also the rest of your family.

**DAY 1**

Juice your first 32oz (1 liter) of apple juice. If you chose to use sour/tart cherry juice, prepare 8oz (240ml). Don't drink the juice in one go. Drink it slowly all through the course of the day, a glass about two hours before or after every meal. If it's too sweet or too sour for you, dilute it in water. However do remember to brush your teeth because the malic acid can be damaging to your dental health.

This is also the day you begin your healthy diet. Eat your foods as whole and as natural as possible and avoid refined sugar, alcohol and food from animal sources. Consume your food warm rather than ice-cold to ease the digestive process. Eat only what is enough to keep you satisfied. Instead of eating two or three meals a day, spread them out into five or six meals. This will keep you fuller for longer and also prevent you from overloading your digestive system.

## DAY 2 – 5

As with Day One, each day you will prepare your quota of juice then drink it in slow sips throughout the day. If you're using apple juice, there's a chance that you might experience some bloating and/or diarrhea. This is a normal reaction because either bile that has been stagnant in your system has been activated and thus needs to be eliminated and also because of the sugar in the apple juice. You can choose to dilute the apple juice with water or switch to sour cherry juice which is less sugary just to see if the symptoms will abate.

Keep your diet as light and as clean as possible by sticking to whole grains, fruits and vegetables and avoiding meat products. This will be especially helpful when you cleanse your colon on Day Three or Four. The Colon Cleanse will clear the path in your colon allowing for easy movement of gallstones and other organic and inorganic substances.

Unlike the Liver Cleanse, a Colon Cleanse does not need extensive preparation. All you need to do is to book an appointment with a certified colon hydrotherapist. Colon hydrotherapists will help you clean your colon by a process known as colon irrigation. It costs a bit of money, but it is a pretty fast method and effective because it is being done by a professional.

If you cannot access or afford a colon irrigation, then a water enema is your next best bet. With a water enema, you can cleanse your colon on your own in the comfort of your home. The process involves introducing water into the colon via the anus for fast intestinal cleaning. It rarely takes more than fifteen minutes. Enema Bags are available in most drug stores. Make sure to get the instructions on how to conduct a water enema safely from your chemist.

## DAY 6

You will be beginning the overnight flush on this evening so you need to start preparing for it right from when you wake up. Unlike the other days, drink ALL of your regular quota of apple or tart cherry juice before mid-morning. Of all the other days, this is when it is most important to maintain a light and clean diet. Protein foods will use up the bile that is critical for the elimination of gallstones and the success of the Liver Cleanse. Do not fast because it will inhibit bile secretion. What you need to do is to strike a balance between foods that will inspire bile production but not use it all up.

Have a light breakfast free of sweeteners, spices, milk, oils or meat. For lunch stick with a light vegetarian meal. Do not use regular salt to flavor it, instead use unrefined sea salt and if you can avoid it, do not cook with any oil other than a small quantity of olive oil.

Your last meal of the day should occur at or before two p.m. then prepare yourself for the overnight flush.

# Chapter 4 :
# The Overnight Flush Step-by-Step

The overnight flush will take approximately nineteen hours (from 5.30 p.m. of Day 6 to 12.30 p.m. of the next day) which includes eight hours of sleep. Below are the steps necessary for conducting an overnight flush organized according to the time they should occur. If you want this process to be a success do not deviate from the set guidelines.

**5.30 p.m.**

In thirty minutes you will be starting the liver cleanse itself. Prepare the Epsom salt and water mixture. As stated in the ingredients, you need 4 tablespoons of Epsom salt and 24oz (710ml) of water. Mix it ALL then divide into four serving portions. You should use sealed containers/bottles instead of glasses to prevent any residue from settling in any of the portions. Keep your portions at room temperature.

**6.00 p.m.**

Drink your first serving of the Epsom salt & water mixture. The best way to drink it is in just one go to prevent gagging. However if you're having a hard time doing it that you can drink *a few* sips of water with a bit of lemon added in to minimize the taste. Afterwards brush your teeth to eliminate both the alkali and the taste. Don't drink any more water until at least fifteen minutes have passed. You also need to set out whichever citrus fruit you chose (be it lemons, grapefruits or oranges) in preparation for juicing about three and a half hours from now.

## 8.00 p.m.

Drink your second serving of the Epsom salt & water mixture. As previously, drink it all in one go if you can and brush your teeth afterwards. Don't drink any more water until at least fifteen minutes have passed.

## 9.30 p.m.

By now you should've had your first bowel movement. If you haven't it's probably because of the colon cleanse you did. However if you didn't do a colon cleanse, then consider performing a water enema right now. If your gallstones are larger, they need a clearer path to travel through and a colon cleanse could help.

## 9.45 p.m.

Remember the citrus fruits you set out? Wash them thoroughly to remove any germs or residue. Make sure your hands are clean too because you're going to be extracting their juice by hand. Squeeze into the measuring jar until you have 6oz (180ml) of juice. Once you've extracted enough juice, mix it with 4oz (120ml) of olive oil (or whatever substitute you chose) in a glass jar. Lid the jar, close tightly and then shake until the blend appears watery.

## 10.00 p.m.

Drink the citrus-olive oil blend in one go. However, if you still feel like going to the bathroom, postpone drinking the blend till the urge passes (could be about ten or fifteen minutes later). Some people have a hard time drinking the citrus-oil blend. Though it is best to take it on its own, you can use a little honey in between sips to sweeten the mix.

## 10.05 p.m.

Immediately after drinking the blend go to your bedroom. Turn the lights off and lie down on the bed on your back. Your head should be propped up by two pillows to aid in the movement of the blend to your liver. Stay in the position for approximately twenty minutes. Don't talk or stand up until these twenty minutes are up, unless you need to go to the bathroom. Otherwise save all your energy for cleansing your liver. Do not drink any water until at least two hours later because you want the oil and citrus to do their work and water will interfere with this process.

## 10.20 p.m.

Now you can move to your usual sleep position as long as it is not lying on your stomach. Stay in bed until you fall asleep unless it's to go to the bathroom. If you do have bowel movement, you might notice small gallstones at this time. The gallstones come in a range of colors from pea-green, tan, dark green, red, white to black. Do not be alarmed to see things other than gallstones e.g. parasites or worms released. This is a cleansing process therefore it will eliminate anything that is obstructing your liver and colon.

## 6.00 a.m.

The moment you wake up drink a glass of warm water. You may wake up feeling a little bit sluggish or nauseous. This is just a sign that you body has been hard at work over the night and the feeling will probably pass by mid-morning. However if it is debilitating take some aloe vera juice to soothe your stomach.

**6.15 a.m.**

Drink the third portion of your Epsom salt-water mix. Even if you feel like going to sleep, resist the impulse. Instead remain upright. Taking a walk or doing your normal household chores may make this process much easier. It may also help you get your energy up and ready you to start the day. Don't drink water until at least fifteen minutes later.

**8.00 a.m.**

Drink the fourth portion of your Epsom salt-water mix. This is your last portion of this blend and we're drawing to an end of overnight flush. As with the other portions try to drink it as quickly as possible and in one go. Do not drink any water until at least fifteen minutes. You should expect a series of watery bowel movements throughout the morning – maybe even up to the afternoon. Most people report fifteen to twenty evacuations of organic and inorganic residue mixed with gallstones. As explained before the gallstones come in a variety of shapes, colors and sizes.

**10.00 a.m.**

You can now take your first meal of the day. However don't get too excited, it's a light meal. Squeeze some fresh juice – whether it is made of citrus or whatever fruits you prefer – and drink. You haven't eaten since last night and your digestive system has undergone an overhaul so you can't just stuff it immediately with solids. Food needs to be introduced slowly starting with liquid nutrition.

**11.30 a.m.**

Now you can introduce some solids into your diet but don't go crazy. A bowl of fresh fruit should be enough. Having an apple, a banana or an avocado should help hold you until your next meal.

**12.30 p.m.**

This is your first 'real' meal of the day. By 'real' I mean that you can include some cooked food in the meal. Make sure the meal is vegetarian and contains limited or no fat.

**IN THE EVENING**

By evening you should be feeling your first signs of revitalization. As with your lunch-time meal, keep your evening meal light and vegetarian.

After three days you can reintroduce meat but keep it limited and white because most meats contain 'bad' fat. You have just revamped your system to get rid of this 'bad' fat so keeping it as clean as you possibly should be your priorities.

# Chapter 5 :
# The Results

The Liver Cleanse is like hitting the refresh button on your computer. Everything speeds up and suddenly you begin to realize the capabilities of your system that had been hidden by whatever obstructions were slowing it down. Most people experience almost immediate relief in their digestive system. Any previous bloating or abdominal pains cause by unfiltered waste disappear.

You will also feel more revitalized and energetic. Because your liver has been unclogged, it is better able to process the nutrients vital in keeping your energy up and purifying your blood. Your performance at work and at home will nominally increase. The appearance of your skin will become softer and smooth as other organs begin to reflect the changes in the state of your liver.

Any allergies you had before will probably lessen or in some cases disappear for good. If you're trying to lose weight and doing all the right things including eating healthy and exercising, you'll most likely start seeing the results of your efforts now. The benefits you will get just from the overnight flush are immense. You will get emotional, physical and mental rejuvenation that can only come from having a cleaner system.

However just because you are experiencing these immense changes, that does not mean that the process is over, Two or three days after the Liver Cleanse, you will need to perform another Colon Cleanse to get rid of any lingering residue. After about three or four weeks you'll need to perform another Liver Cleanse. Why?

Well, one flush is seldom enough to get rid of all the gallstones in your liver especially if this is the first time you're doing it. You'll need to perform it after every three or four weeks till you see no gallstones during bowel movements. Don't avoid it because it seems inconvenient. Your body will not thank you for it.

A normal reaction of the body is that when it realizes that a cleaning process is taking place it will dump any other hidden toxins it was holding on to. This is why when you're sick, the first few days after you begin taking the drugs you'll feel a bit sicker. The body is releasing even the sickness it had hidden. If you had headaches before the colon cleanse or other symptoms they will reappear, though to a lesser extent. Doing another Liver Cleanse to eliminate lingering gallstones will get rid of them for good.

Two or three back to back Liver Cleanses separated by three or four weeks should be enough to completely revamp your system. Once you're gallstone-free you can reduce your Liver Cleanse to just once every six to eight months.

## WHAT IF IT DOESN'T WORK?

If you did not follow all the instructions as laid out the Liver Cleanse may not work. Ask yourself;

1. Did I use all the ingredients as prescribed and not try to substitute them?

2. Did I maintain a clean and light diet all through the period leading up to the overnight flush?

3. During the overnight flush did I follow each step precisely as outlined?

4. Did I do a Colon Cleanse two or three days before and after the Liver Cleanse?

If you answered 'No' to any of these questions, then wait for three to four weeks then perform the colon cleanse again but this time as prescribed.

There are some people who will follow all the instructions and still not get any results. In such a case the most probable reason is that you have denser than average gallstones that are severely congesting your bile ducts. The Malic Acid in the apple-juice or tart cherry juice was not enough to soften them over the six day processes. You need a stronger gallstone breaker.

Taking twenty drops of Chanca Piedra three times daily for three weeks preceding your next Liver Cleanse has been shown to be especially effective at this task. Your local natural food store should have Chanca Piedra stocked. If you cannot find it then use three tablespoons of undiluted and unsweetened lemon juice fifteen to thirty minutes before breakfast every day for the three weeks preceding your next attempt at a liver cleanse.

Do not give up just because of one failed attempt. Your commitment to this process will be rewarding. In just a few weeks, you will be able to look and feel younger.

# Chapter 6 :
# After The Liver Cleanse

Now that you have a cleaner liver, you need to keep it that way. Nobody wants to go back to the situation that caused the gallstones in the first place and the unpleasant symptoms that came with it. Keeping your liver clean isn't a hard task. It just requires a bit of a lifestyle change that will keep you looking and feeling good.

**WATCH YOUR DIET**

The most important component to keeping your liver healthy is maintaining a healthy diet. A diet rich in whole grains, vegetables, fruits and good oils (Omega 3) is the best for your body. The high fiber content in these foods will make the digestive process much easier for the liver and thus keep it working at optimum capacity.

Three or four days after the Liver Cleanse you can reintroduce animal products into your meal. However even then try to keep away from red meats. The problem with red meats (beef, lamb, goat etc) is that they contain a lot of Low Density Lipoprotein (LDL) or 'bad' fat which is hard to filter out of the system. Because of the way most livestock are raised these days, it often also contains a lot of toxic additives that affect the liver functions. Where you can, opt for poultry or fish instead of a red meat.

Replace processed sugars with healthier options like honey and regular salt with sea salt. These options contain more nutrients that will improve your general health system. Replace your regular coffee with a blend of lemon, ginger and warm water. Ginger will mimic the actions of coffee to awaken your system while lemon is extremely effective in breaking stones. With these changes in your diet you should be able to minimize the accumulation of toxins and the formation of new gallstones.

## EXERCISE REGULARLY

Exercise is a critical component in maintaining your liver and overall body health. The human body is different from machines. The more you use it, the better it gets at its job. You need at least thirty minutes of vigorous exercise each day. You don't even have to join a gym. A brisk walk around your neighborhood, a basketball game or even heavy household chores like moping or gardening are ways to keep your body at optimum condition. Exercise has the added benefit of inducing 'happy' endorphins in the body which will reduce stress. When balanced with seven to eight hours of sleep each day, your days will become much more pleasant.

## AVOID ALCOHOL, SMOKING & DRUGS

Nothing ruins a Liver Cleanse like alcohol, smoking and drugs. These three monsters contain dizzying proportions of toxins. Alcohol is notorious for causing fatty liver, hepatitis and cirrhosis. When drunk, alcohol is absorbed into the blood stream and first goes through the liver for breaking down into water and carbon-dioxide. The liver can only deal with a certain amount of alcohol per hour. When you drink alcohol faster than your liver can process, the level of alcohol in your bloodstream rises. That highly coveted 'high' feeling is actually the liver's way of warning you that it is overwhelmed. And when the liver is overwhelmed, the end result is it functioning at less than optimum capacity.

Smoking on the other hand ages the liver. The liver needs oxygen to perform its functions and this it usually extracts from the blood. Cigarette smoke inhibits the red blood cells capacity to transport oxygen to all organs, including the liver. Little oxygen means oxidative stress in the liver and eventual aging because this state damages the liver cells and fibrosis. When alcohol and smoking are taken in combination, you're basically signing your liver's death warrant.

So just don't!

**AVOID EXPOSURE TO TOXINS**

Most people assume that toxins only come from moldy walls and insecticides (and they do) but have you checked the lotions, deodorant and make up you use lately? Look at your favorite makeup and see what components have been used to make it. As we said before, anything you eat, inhale or absorb through the skin is headed straight for the liver so you need to make sure it's going to build it not harm it.

Some of these lotions have additives that you'd be shocked to realize you're putting on your skin. Read the labels carefully on everything you use on your skin to see what ingredients they have. Do your research to see what the point of each of those ingredients is and if they have any side-effects. Once you've found a product that you feel is completely safe stick to it and avoid experimenting. Or better yet find ways to make your own natural lotions, deodorants and other skin and/or odor enhancers.

Don't even try procedures like tanning and bleaching. You may look good now, but ten to twenty years from now is when you'll realize the kind of damage you are doing not only to your skin but also to your liver.

## FREQUENT LIVER CLEANSE

After the last batch of gallstones has been eliminated from your liver via the back-to-back Liver Cleanses, every six to eight months you need to do another cleanse. The reason for this is that despite our best efforts we are only human. Sometimes we slip back into bad lifestyle habits and our bodies catch the flack for these slips. Instead of feeling guilty for not being able to maintain a clean diet all the time, just schedule a cleanse to reboot your system. But don't make slipping a habit – your liver can only take so much.

## GET CONSTANT MEDICAL CHECK UPS

Despite our best efforts to take care of ourselves, sometimes the body just has a mind of its own. It's no good to take care of your liver and ignore the rest of your system where something else could be going wrong. The only way to keep a close eye on the rest of your body is to schedule regular appointments with your doctor even when it seems like nothing is wrong. Some of the tests you need to take include tests for cholesterol, high blood pressure, STIs and cancer. With regular checkups you should be able to net any other parts of your system that are going rogue.

# Conclusion

Thank you for taking the time to read The Natural Liver Detox Cleanse: a proven 7 day program to cleanse your liver, lose weight and reclaim your health. I trust that this guide will help you perform a liver cleanse easily, safely and successful.

Everyone should do a Liver Cleanse at least once in their lifetime if not more. The benefits that come with it are incredible. Think of your body as a car that requires frequent servicing to increase its capacity to perform. Like servicing, the Liver Cleanse will energize and revitalize you, and ultimately increase your life expectancy. If you follow the instructions for both the preparation week and the overnight flush, precisely as prescribed, you'll be well on your way to better health.

If this guide was helpful to you, please share it with your family and friends, and introduce them to better health. Of course not everyone will be open-minded to the process but none of the ingredients used are in any way harmful and the results afterwards speak for themselves.

Thank you and good luck!

# Bonus

# THE NATURAL FATTY LIVER CURE

## Healthy Recipes That Support Your Liver

### R. Huntington

© 2014 Copyright.
Text copyright reserved. R. Huntington

The contents of this book may not be reproduced, duplicated or transmitted without direct written permission from the author.

Disclaimer : all attempts have been made by the author to provide factual and accurate content. No responsibility will be taken by the author for any damages caused by misuse of the content described in this book. The content of this book has been derived from various sources. Please consult a licensed professional before attempting any techniques outlined in this book.

# Table of Contents

**Introduction** ............................................................. 66

**Breakfast: Getting Starting on the Right Foot** ............................................................. 68

Recipe 1: A Delicious Cereal that is Liver Friendly, Ready in Minutes and Joy to Eat .................................. 68

Recipe 2: A Caramelized Baked Oats and Apple Treat that You Will Want Seconds Of ........................... 70

Recipe 3: A Smoothie that Should be Part of Your Morning Routine ..................................................... 72

Recipe 4: Another Breakfast Smoothie that is Liver Friendly and Flavorful ............................................ 73

Recipe 5: Liver friendly Breakfast Bars that You can Grab and Go or Use as a 'Go To' Snack Throughout the Day ........................................................ 75

**Lunch: Adding the Protein Back In to Your Day** 78

Recipe 1: Rainbow Trout Meatballs – Full of Everything that You Look Forward to at Lunch ............ 78

Recipe 2: Pad Thai Gets a Spring Roll Makeover that is Easy to Make and Absolutely Delectable to Eat ......... 81

Recipe 3: Salmon Hot Pot Loaded with Veggie Goodness – Both Yum and Satisfying .......................... 85

Recipe 4: Mediterranean Style Lettuce Wraps that Pack a Potent Flavor Punch ...... 87

**Dinner:** .................................................. 89

Recipe 1: A Couscous, Cannellini Bean, Apple, and Brussels Sprouts Dish that will have the Entire Family Asking for Seconds ............... 89

Recipe 2: Light and Spicy Dinner - Turkey Chili ............ 92

Recipe 3: Another Mediterranean Delight: Healthy Baked Falafels with a Zesty Sauce ............ 94

**Conclusion** ................................................. 97

# Introduction

Hi there! I am glad you decided to pick up this book to use the dietary information and recipes in it (mostly recipes) to help heal and even reverse the effects of fatty Liver Disease. Fatty Liver Disease or Non-Alcoholic Liver Disease has been strongly linked to the rise in the obesity epidemic. For sufferers the amount, type, and quality of food consumed on a regular basis is the leading reason behind developing a 'fatty liver'.

A fatty liver is basically a liver that has more than 5% of fat in it. This means that the liver is damaged and is not working at its best. This is also a warning because if precautions and lifestyle changes are not made, then this condition to deteriorate further resulting in more serious health complication and even fatalities. The lifestyle choices that we cause this condition to recess include holistic living and a healthy diet regimen. Reversing the effects of years' worth of bad eating habits will not happen overnight or even in a few weeks or months. This transition has to become a way of living and eating for the sufferer in order to achieve long term success against the disease.

This cookbook will focus only on the eating habits that will help in recovery. Learning to cook delicious, tempting food, all the while caring for your liver will make the journey of your recovery and beyond not just a successful, but also a pleasurable one. You will start seeing healthy, good for you, but not so great tasting foods transform into delectable dishes that you will look forward to indulging in.

This cookbook does not give an exhaustive list of recipes because that is not the aim here; the aim here is to get you to see nutritious food in a different perspective. Once you familiarize with the ingredients and recipe patterns than you can start to experiment with new recipes or adapt old favorites to this new way of healthy eating. We are literally following the saying, *"give a man a fish, you feed him for a day. Teach him how to catch fish and you feed him for a lifetime."* Learning to adapt and experiment according to your needs and tastes is an infinitely better way to start this journey of recovery than any other is.

Don't you agree?

# Breakfast:
# Getting Starting on the Right Foot

Cleansing your liver is most effectively done through a better breakfast than any other meal. Starting the day right with the right liver strength boosting foods is important in order to keep the momentum going throughout the day. A liver friendly breakfast should be high in good carbohydrates, like whole wheat bread and cereal. Adding fruit and vegetable is also great. Limiting protein and salt intake at breakfast is also crucial for a good liver cleanse. Let us look at a few recipes that will give the right start to your day, use these as inspiration to start building your own recipes. Using your favorite flavor combinations.

**Recipe 1: A Delicious Cereal that is Liver Friendly, Ready in Minutes and Joy to Eat**

*Preparation Time (approx.): 8 - 10 minutes*

*Cooking Time: 0 minutes*

*Servings: 1*

*Ingredient List for Cereal*

    Quinoa – ¾ cup (cooked or leftover from before)

    Mixed Nuts – 1 tablespoon (coarsely chopped)

    Soy or Almond Milk – 1 cup + 2 tablespoons for serving (You can use skim milk or rice milk too)

    Sunflower Seeds – 1 tablespoon (toasted)

Beets – 1 small (finely grated)

Cinnamon Powder – 1 teaspoon

Dates – 1 tablespoon (chopped)

Pomegranate – 2 tablespoons (if in season, otherwise leave it out or replace with seasonal fruit)

## *Steps*

1. Start by pacing the cooked quinoa at the bottom of a serving bowl.
2. Heat the milk over low heat so that it becomes slightly warm to the touch but not hot.
3. Add the mixed nuts, sunflower seeds, grated beets, chopped dates, and pomegranate.
4. Pour the warm milk over the bowl full of ingredients and mix well.
5. Sprinkle with cinnamon power and add the cold splash of milk right before serving or eating. Enjoy your crunchy, tasty, liver friendly breakfast.

## Recipe 2: A Caramelized Baked Oats and Apple Treat that You Will Want Seconds Of

*Preparation Time (approx.): 5 – 8 minutes*

*Cooking Time: 45 – 50 minutes*

*Servings: 3*

*Ingredient List for Baked Apple and Oats Cereal*

- Steel Cut Oats – 1 cup
- Apples – 3 medium (cut into wedges)
- Maple Syrup – 3 tablespoons (organic)
- Ginger – ½" inch (fresh, ground to paste)
- Chia Seeds – 1 tablespoon
- Pumpkin Seeds – ¼ cup
- Sesame seeds – ½ tablespoon (toasted)
- Sea Salt – a pinch
- Cinnamon Powder – 1 teaspoon
- Nutmeg – 1 teaspoon (freshly grated)
- Water – 3 cups (boiling)

**Steps**

1. Preheat oven to 375 F and make ready a casserole dish for baking.

2. Using a medium sized, heavy bottom skillet over medium heat, toast the steel cut oats.

3. As the oats just start to turn color, add the cinnamon powder, and nutmeg and roast for a couple of more minutes or until the oats are fragrant from the spices and toasted.

4. Bring the water to a boil on a separate burner.

5. Empty the contents of the skillet into the casserole dish. Sprinkle the Chia seeds, pumpkin seeds, salt, and toasted sesame seeds on top. Combine all the ingredient well.

6. Place the apple on top of all the other ingredients in the casserole dish and pour the maple syrup over them, saving half or a quarter of the syrup for bushing later.

7. Lastly, pour the boiling water over all the ingredients and place in the oven.

8. Bake for 40 minutes, but after 30 minutes take the dish out and pour the remaining maple syrup over the apples and all the other ingredients to force further caremalization.

9. Bake for another 10 minutes and serve warm.

## Recipe 3: A Smoothie that Should be Part of Your Morning Routine

*Preparation Time (approx.): 5 – 8 minutes*

*Cooking Time: 0 minutes*

*Servings: 1*

*Ingredient List for Liver Cleansing Smoothie*

- Beets – 2 medium (peeled)
- Ginger – ½" fresh
- Lemon – 1 medium (peeled)
- Apple – 1 medium
- Cilantro – ¼ cup (chopped)
- Chia Seeds – ½ tablespoons
- Salt – 1 pinch
- Black pepper – 1 sprinkle

### Steps

1. Start by juicing the beets, ginger, lemon, cilantro, and apple together.
2. Blend the juice with chia seeds in a blender. Sprinkle a little salt n pepper on top (optional) and drink up!

## Recipe 4: Another Breakfast Smoothie that is Liver Friendly and Flavorful

*Preparation Time (approx.): 5 – 8 minutes*

*Cooking Time: 0 minutes*

*Servings: 1*

*Ingredient List for Liver Cleansing Smoothie 2*

- Beets – 1 medium (peeled, halved)
- Red Apples – 2 medium (pith removed, halved)
- Orange – 1 medium (peeled)
- Carrots – 3 medium (peeled)
- Ginger – ½" fresh
- Turmeric Powder – ½ teaspoon (turmeric has a metallic taste so you can start with even lesser turmeric and add more in as you get used to the taste)
- Flax Seeds – 1 tablespoon

### Steps

1. Start by juicing the beet, red apples, orange, carrots, and ginger together.
2. Blend the juice roughly with turmeric powder and flax seeds in a blender. Drink immediately for keep in a cool

place for a few hours. Best to drink it immediately because the antioxidants are the most potent when the juices are freshest.

## Recipe 5: Liver friendly Breakfast Bars that You can Grab and Go or Use as a 'Go To' Snack Throughout the Day

*Preparation Time (approx.): 7 – 9 minutes*

*Cooking Time: 45 – 50 minutes*

*Servings: 8 bars*

*Ingredient List of Almond Bars*

- Almonds – ¾ cup (lightly toasted, with skin)
- Cashew Nuts – ¾ cup (lightly toasted)
- Coconut Flakes – 1½ cups (lightly toasted)
- Maple Syrup – ½ cup (organic)
- Sesame Seeds – 1 teaspoon (toasted)
- Sunflower Seeds – 1 tablespoon (toasted)
- Raisins – ½ tablespoon (chopped)
- Water – 3 tablespoons
- Sea Salt – a pinch

## Steps

1. Start by Preheating the oven to 325 F. Make ready a 8 x 8 inch square baking pan by lining it with parchment paper.

2. In a medium sized, heavy bottomed pot, add the maple syrup, water, and a pinch of salt. Place over medium high heat and heat until the mixture starts to boil. At this point, lower the heat so that the mixture comes down to a simmer.

3. Do not cover the liquid and let it reduce to a thick consistency similar to dense honey. This should take 25 to 30 minutes.

4. As the liquid is reducing place the toasted almonds, cashew nuts, coconut flakes, sesame seeds, sunflower seeds, and chopped raisins in a medium sized mixing bowl and mix well.

5. As the liquid is reduced enough to a honey like consistency, pour it over the ingredients in the mixing bowl and using a spoon, mix well so that all the nuts, seeds, flakes, ad raising are well coated.

6. Transfer this mixture onto the readied baking pan, making sure that all ingredients are evenly distributed.

7. Place a parchment sheet on top of the mixture and using a wide faced wooden spoon or a rolling pin (if it fits in the pan) to press down on the ingredients firmly. Press down as hard as you can until you feel there is no more space left to between the ingredient layers and they are as compact as they can be.

8. Remove the top parchment paper and let the bars cool down at room temperature.

9. Once cool to the touch, empty the pan onto a flat surface or a cutting board and using a sharp knife cut the block into 8 to 10 rectangular bars. Let the individual bars completely cool down and harden.

10. Store the bars in an airtight container for later or enjoy immediately.

# Lunch:
# Adding the Protein Back In to Your Day

Lunch typically offers more variety of foods because white meats are allowed at lunch along with different protein packed legumes. Fatty Liver sufferers are recommended to restrict their protein intake to help heal and repair their livers. However, protein is still the building block of cells in our bodies and consuming good proteins are just as important as eliminating bad (or tougher to digest) proteins out of your diet. Always opt for meat option that are either white or are very lean. Legumes are an excellent protein source because not only are they versatile in cooking techniques and flavors, but the plant based protein they provide is the gentler on the liver.

## Recipe 1: Rainbow Trout Meatballs – Full of Everything that You Look Forward to at Lunch

*Preparation Time (approx.): 8 – 10 minutes*

*Cooking Time: 30 – 35 minutes*

*Servings: 5*


*Ingredient List for Meatballs*

- Rainbow Trout – 1½ pounds (steamed or broiled, shredded)

- Eggs – 3 medium (scrambled but not overcooked)

- Red Onion – 1 small (finely chopped)

- Garlic – 2 cloves (minced)

Cilantro – ¼ cup (roughly chopped)

Panko Bread Crumbs – 1 tablespoon

Sea Salt – to taste

Black Pepper – to taste (freshly ground)

*Ingredient List for Salsa*

Tomatoes – 2 cups (seasonal, deseeded, chopped)

Cilantro – ½ cup (chopped)

Garlic – 6 cloves (finely chopped)

Yellow Onion – 1 small (chopped)

Lime Juice – 1 tablespoon (freshly squeezed, if possible)

Jalapeño – 1 medium (finely chopped)

Sea Salt – to taste

## **Steps**

*For Preparing the Meatballs:* Start by preheating the oven to 350 F and make ready a baking tray by lining with aluminum foil or parchment paper.

1. In a medium sized bowl, add the shredded rainbow trout, garlic, onions, cilantro, and Panko bread crumbs. Mix well.

2. Now add the semi cooked scrambled eggs to the same bowl and combine well.

3. Season with sea salt and pepper according to taste and now bring the mixture together using your hands.

4. Once the mixture start coming together make 1" to 1½" inch meatballs. You should have more or less twenty meatballs.

5. Place the meatballs on the readied baking tray and bake for 30 minutes. Or until the outside becomes golden brown.

6. *For Preparing the Salsa:* To create the salsa for dipping the meatballs simple combine all the ingredients i.e. tomatoes, cilantro, garlic, onion, jalapeño, lime juice, and sea salt in an airtight container.

7. Combine well and let rest in the fridge for as long as possible. Overnight is best to get the most depth in flavors.

8. Serve the chilled salsa with hot, freshly baked or heated meatballs for a delicious and healthy lunch.

## Recipe 2: Pad Thai Gets a Spring Roll Makeover that is Easy to Make and Absolutely Delectable to Eat

*Preparation Time (approx.): 5 – 10 minutes*

*Cooking Time: 10 – 15 minutes*

*Servings: 3*

*Ingredient List for Tofu Marinade*

- Tofu – ½ block (cut into 4" long strips)
- Rice Wine Vinegar – 1/8 cup
- Apple Cider Vinegar – 1/8 cup
- Warm Water – 1 cup
- Chicken or Beef Stock – ¼ cup
- Garlic – 2 cloves (minced)
- Red Chili Flakes – a pinch
- Sea Salt – to taste
- Black Pepper – to taste (freshly ground)

*Ingredient List for Spring Rolls*

- Rice Noodles – ½ cup
- Coconut Oil – I tablespoon (room temperature)

Spring Onions – 1 bunch (cut into strips)

Carrots – 2 medium (cut into strips)

Celery – ½ Stalk (cut into strips)

Leeks – 1 medium (cut into strips)

Sun Dried Tomatoes – 2 (cut into strips)

Peanuts – 2 tablespoons (crushed)

Basil – 1 tablespoon (chopped, fresh)

Cilantro – 1/6 cup (chopped)

Rice Paper – 4 to 6

*Ingredient List for Pad Thai Sauce*

Chicken or Beef Stock – 2 tablespoons

Garlic – 1 clove (minced)

Lime Juice – ½ lime (freshly squeezed)

Agave Nectar – 1 tablespoon

Sesame Oil – ¼ teaspoon

Red Chili Flakes – a pinch (optional)

*Ingredient List for Peanut Sauce*

Chicken or Beef Stock – 2 tablespoons

Peanut Butter – 2 tablespoons (smooth)

Garlic – ½ clove (minced)

Sesame Seeds – ½ teaspoon

Sriracha – 1/8 teaspoon

Agave Nectar – 2 teaspoons

Lime Juice – 1 teaspoon (freshly squeezed)

Hot Water - 2½ tablespoons

## *Steps*

1. *For Marinating the Tofu:* To begin take a medium mixing bowl, add all the marinade ingredients i.e. rice wine vinegar, apple cider vinegar, warm water, chicken stock, garlic, red chili flakes, except one – the tofu. Combine the ingredients using a whisk.

2. Once combined pour the marinade into a shallow dish. Simply place your tofu stripes inside the marinade and let the flavors permeate into one another. Marinade overnight if possible, if not, even a two hour marinating should be enough.

3. *For Making the Pad Thai Sauce:* Take a medium mixing bowl, and add all the ingredients for the Pad Thai sauce i.e. stock, garlic, lime juice, agave nectar, sesame oil, and red chili flakes using a whisk.

4. Begin by cooking the whole wheat pasta by bringing salted water to a boil and adding the pasta to it. Cook

until al-dente (simply meaning that it still has a little bite and is not completely cooked through). Drain and let the pasta cool.

5. *For Making the Peanut Sauce:* Take a small mixing bowl, add all the ingredients for the peanut sauce i.e. stock, peanut butter, garlic, sesame seeds, sriracha, agave nectar, lime juice, and hot water. Whisk together to combine well and set aside.

6. *For Making the Spring Rolls:* Start by cooking your noodles in salted, boiling water according to the manufacturer's directions on the box. If you are making the pasta from scratch cook the pasta to an al dente.

7. Once cooked, toss the same noodles in the pad Thai sauce and coat well.

8. In a medium sized skillet, sauté the tofu on medium heat in coconut oil. Make sure that the tofu is browned on all sides.

9. Using hot water, soak and soften the rice paper in a bowl to make it edible.

10. Assemble the healthy spring rolls, but placing the rice paper at the bottom and laying all the ingredients one by one on top. Do not forget your favorite vegetables.

11. Serve or eat with the peanut sauce prepared earlier for a final boost in flavor right before we consume the food. Enjoy!

## Recipe 3: Salmon Hot Pot Loaded with Veggie Goodness – Both Yum and Satisfying

*Preparation Time (approx.): 5 – 10 minutes*

*Cooking Time: 15 – 20 minutes*

*Servings: 2*


*Ingredient List for Hot Pot*

- Salmon – 2 Fillets (3 – 4 pounds each, skinless)
- Shiitake Mushrooms – ¼ cup (dried)
- Baby Spinach – 1 cup
- Cabbage – 1 cup
- Carrots – 1 cup (cut into matchsticks)
- White Miso – to taste
- Sea Salt – to taste
- Black Pepper – to taste (freshly ground)
- Chicken or Vegetable Stock – 4 cups (low fat and low sodium preferred)

## Steps

1. Preheat oven to 300 F. Ready a casserole dish by spreading the miso over the bottom of the ceramic pot. You can be as generous with miso as you want, but if you feel that the 'fish' taste is too strong, use it sparingly just make sure you spread it over the entire bottom.

2. Take a medium sized, heavy bottom saucepan and place it over medium heat. Add the vegetable or chicken stock to it and bring to a boil.

3. As the stock gets heated, place the salmon fillets, shiitake mushrooms, baby spinach, cabbage, and carrots into the ceramic pot that has been layered with miso.

4. Pour all the hot stock over the vegetables and fish and cover with lid.

5. Season with sea salt and pepper, but use salt as sparingly as possible to keep the sodium content low.

6. Place the pot in the oven and let it cook for 15 to 20 minutes or until the fish fillets are just starting to fall apart.

7. Serve immediately or keep in an airtight container after the soup has cooled down slightly for later in the day or the week.

## Recipe 4: Mediterranean Style Lettuce Wraps that Pack a Potent Flavor Punch

*Preparation Time (approx.): 10 – 12 minutes*

*Cooking Time: 8 – 10 minutes*

*Servings: 4*


*Ingredient List for Hot Pot*

- Bulgur Wheat – 2 cups (cooked)
- Extra Virgin Olive Oil – 2 tablespoons
- Tomatoes – 3 medium (seasonal, deseeded, diced)
- French Onion – ¼ cup (diced)
- Cucumber – 1 medium (diced)
- Boston Lettuce – 8 leaves
- Feta Cheese – 1 tablespoon (crumbled)
- Lemon Juice – 2 tablespoons
- Sea Salt – to taste
- Black Pepper – to taste (freshly ground)
- Parsley – 2 cups (chopped)
- Mint – 2 tablespoons (chopped)
- Water – 2 cups

## Steps

1. Begin by cooking the bulgur in 2 cups of boiling water in a large saucepan. Boil until the bulgur is cooked or for 5 minutes in the boiling water. Remove the saucepan from heat, cover it and let rest for 15 to 20 minutes or until the pot is cooled enough to touch.

2. Drain the excess water through a cauldron and return the cooked bulgur to a medium sized, airtight bowl. Close the lid and refrigerate for a couple of hours or until the bulgur has chilled.

3. Take a large mixing bowl and add all the vegetables i.e. tomatoes, French onions, cucumber, and the herbs (mint and parsley) to it. Mix well

4. Once the bulgurm, is chilled transfer it to the large mixing bowl with the vegetables and herbs and combine well.

5. In a smaller mixing bowl, add the extra virgin olive oil and mix it with the lemon juice, sea salt, and pepper using a whisk.

6. Pour this olive oil and lemon juice mixture over the bulgur, vegetable, and herb mixture and combine well using a wooden spoon.

7. Place lettuce leaves onto the serving dish and ladle ¼ or ½ of the Mediterranean stuffing (called Tabbouleh) onto each leaf.

8. Garnish with a bit of crumbled Feta each and enjoy.

## Dinner:

Dinner as is our societal norm should be both comforting and hearty. There are exceptions, but most of us like to come home to a satisfying big meal. For Fatty Liver sufferers there is absolutely no limit on the amount of food they can consume at dinner. However, choosing lighter options like steamed or roasted rather than fried food is important. Choosing leaner cuts of meat also helps as does adding vegetables as a salad or a side to your main meal. Replacing skim milk and low fat dairy with full fat milk and dairy also helps heal the liver. If you are starting to feel restricted in your choices, do not. Just read the recipes below to find out how much flavor and food you can pack into liver loving foods.

### Recipe 1: A Couscous, Cannellini Bean, Apple, and Brussels Sprouts Dish that will have the Entire Family Asking for Seconds

*Preparation Time (approx.): 12 – 15 minutes*

*Cooking Time: 20 to 25 minutes*

*Servings: 6*

*Ingredient List for Couscous*

    Couscous – 1 cup (uncooked)

    Extra Virgin Olive Oil – 2 tablespoons

    Brussels Sprouts – 3 cups (chopped)

    Apple – 1 medium (diced)

Cannellini Beans – 1 cup (drain ad rinse one 8 oz. can)

Vegetable or Chicken Broth – 1¼ cup (low fat, low sodium)

Balsamic Vinegar – ¼ cup and 2 tablespoons separate (low sodium)

French Onion – 1 medium (chopped)

Pine Nuts – ¼ cup (toasted, crushed)

Italian Seasoning – 1 teaspoon

Sea Salt – to taste

Black Pepper – to taste (freshly ground)

## Steps

1. Start by cooking the couscous in a medium sized, heavy bottomed pot by boiling the vegetable or chicken broth and adding the couscous and sea salt to it. Turn the heat off. Cover and set aside.

2. Take a large, heavy bottomed skillet and place of medium heat. Add the olive oil to it, as it starts to heat up add the onions and cook them over medium heat until they become translucent or for 4 to 5 minutes.

3. Once the onions are done, add the Brussels sprouts and the apple and cook uncovered, stirring occasionally. Cook until the apple start getting tender on the outside or for 10 minutes.

4. Season the onions, Brussels sprouts, and apple with sea salt, pepper, 2 tablespoons of Balsamic vinegar, and the Italian seasoning. Combine well.

5. Add the cannellini beans and combine with the rest of the mixture gently, using a wooden spoon. Cook for a few minutes (4 to 5) or until the beans are completely combined and warmed through.

6. In a small sized, heavy bottom sauce pan on medium heat and add ¼ cup of balsamic vinegar. Bring the vinegar to a boil. Turn the heat to low and let simmer while stirring so that the vinegar takes on thicker, syrup like consistency.

7. To serve layer the couscous at the bottom of the service dish or bowl, ladle over the cannellini bean mixture and pour or drizzle the syrupy balsamic vinegar on top. Garnish with toasted crushed pine nuts and enjoy.

## Recipe 2: Light and Spicy Dinner - Turkey Chili

*Preparation Time (approx.): 20 – 25 minutes*

*Cooking Time: 8 hours*

*Servings: 2*


*Ingredient List for*

    Turkey – 1 pound (ground, extra lean)

    Tomato Sauce – 3¾ cups (low sodium, sugar free)

    Black Beans – 1¾ cups (drained, rinsed)

    Chili Beans – 1 Can (15 oz., un-drained)

    Tomatoes – 1 cup (diced)

    Canned Green Chilies – ¾ cup (slightly drained)

    Bell Peppers – 2 large (sliced in strips)

    French Onion – 1 medium (diced)

    Carrots – 1 cup (peeled, diced)

    Corn – 1 cup (if canned, drain and rinse)

    Garlic – 4 cloves (minced)

    Red Chili Flakes – 1 teaspoon (or reduce if sensitive to heat)

    Cumin Powder – 1 teaspoon

Sea Salt – to taste

Black Pepper – to taste (freshly ground)

**Steps**

1. Begin by taking a large, heavy bottom crockpot and add the ground, raw turkey meat to it. Place over medium heat and brown the meat slightly, stirring constantly.

2. Add Tomato sauce, black beans, chili beans, tomatoes, bell peppers, French onion, carrots, corn kernels, minced garlic, chili flakes, cumin powder and bring to a boil.

3. Once boiled turn the heat to low and let cook for up to 9 hours for best results. You cam turn the heat to low and let it cook slowly for 4 – 5 hours. The object is to get all the vegetables soft and falling apart on touch. Enjoy right away once cooked or store in an airtight jar for later.

## Recipe 3: Another Mediterranean Delight: Healthy Baked Falafels with a Zesty Sauce

*Preparation Time (approx.): 5 – 8 minutes*

*Cooking Time: 18 – 20 minutes*

*Servings: 4*

*Ingredient List for Falafels*

- Chickpeas – 1 cup (drained, rinsed)
- Chickpea Flour – 2 tablespoons
- Semolina – to coat
- French Onion – ½ medium (chopped)
- Garlic – 2 cloves (minced)
- Ginger – ½ inch piece (fresh, paste)
- Cumin Powder – 1 teaspoon
- Cilantro – ½ cup (packed, fresh)
- Sea Salt – to taste
- Black Pepper – to taste (freshly ground)

*Ingredient List for Sauce*

Sesame Seeds – 1½ tablespoon (lightly toasted, ground to paste (tahini))

Dijon Mustard – ½ teaspoon

Sriracha – to taste

Water – 2 tablespoon (room temperature)

**Steps**

1. Begin by preheating the oven to 400 F. Make ready a baking tray by lining it with parchment paper.

2. Now blend the chopped onion, cilantro, and garlic cloves to a paste, using a food processor. As the paste comes together and starts to come away from the walls of the processor and the cumin powder, ginger, sea salt, and pepper. Pulse a few times to combine.

3. Next add to the food processor the chickpeas and again pulse to coarsely blend for a bit of bite and texture. However, if you prefer a smooth texture feel free to blend the chickpeas with the rest of the ingredients and spices until smooth.

4. Transfer the mixture to a large mixing bowl and add the chickpea flour to it. Now stir gently until all the chickpea flour is incorporated.

5. In a small mixing bowl, add the semolina to dip and coat the falafels in before baking.

6. Roll the falafel mixture into balls that are 1" to 1½" inch in diameter. Roll each ball in the semolina to cover completely before placing on the parchment paper. Press the tops of each falafel once you are done placing all of them on the baking tray.

7. Bake until fragrant and golden brown or for 25 minutes. Flip the falafels half way through to cook the bottom similar to the top.

8. As the falafels are baking prepare the sauce by taking a small mixing bowl, and adding the sesame seed paste (tahini), Dijon mustard, sriracha, and the water. Combine well using a whisk.

9. Serve the falafels hot with the spicy sauce and a side of fresh cut vegetables or salad. You can keep the falafels in an airtight box, in the fridge for 5 to 8 days.

# Conclusion

In the end, I wanted to share and reiterate a few pieces of advice that will help you through this journey of healing ad transformation. Disease is rampant in our societies today because of a number of factors but the most common culprit for causing our health woes, is the obesity epidemic. As our waistlines continue to grow so does our chart at the doctors. Joint pain, diabetes, heart diseases, hypertension, kidney disease, liver disease, and many other fatal diseases are all directly linked to abnormal weight gain and obesity.

This is something we have to be aware of and consciously fight at all times. Fighting disease through a better diet will not be a cosmetic solution. It will heal and repair from within giving life to and repairing cells within our bodies that we had not even realized required healing. A healthy diet will build up our body's defenses instead of breaking them down. The best and long lasting cure for liver disease is a good, healthy, liver friendly, diet.

To stick to any diet whether good for you or bad you need the food to be delicious, you need it to tempt you. Eating bland in this world of excess is something only a rare few can accomplish. We need our food to excite us because that is what food does for millions of us everyday. Just because you have a disease does not mean you have to give up eating great tasting food. Through this cookbook and through your own experimentation you can eat to both satisfy and to delight.

I wish you nothing but good health and fortune on this healing journey.

Printed in Great Britain
by Amazon